YOU, ME, COFFEE & TWO DOUGHNUTS LATER

A Conversation About Health & Fitness Between Two Strangers

TALLYSON NEVES

CONTENTS

DISCLAIMER

This is no more than an informative general health-related guide that should be used for educational purposes only. The following guide does not constitute professional medical advice. Please consult a medical or health professional before beginning any exercise, nutrition, or supplementation program. If you choose to engage in any activity or practice described in the following guide, you do so of your own free will, and knowingly and voluntarily accept any and all possible risks. The information which follows in this guide consists of recommendations based on sources and facts, as well as personal and client anecdotal experiences. Much of the information in this work is also taken from the success and failures of many professional and high-level competitors and athletes alike.

ACKNOWLEDGEMENTS

I find starting is the most difficult part of any journey, especially when that journey leads to the creation of something you can uniquely and proudly call yours. You try to shoot for perfection before the journey has begun and will not accept anything less. This leaves you paralyzed, or with me it does at least. You're filled with contradictory feelings: you know all the next steps that should be taken, while at the same time you don't know where to start. And then the thoughts of self-doubt start pouring in. But yet, that longing for the adventure, to create something you can call yours, despite your doubts, won't leave the back of your mind until you tackle it. It's overwhelming.

Those were the feelings I had when I had the idea of writing this book or with any project I've ever taken. The first leap is hard, but thankfully I had the right people in my corner who believed in me and knew I had something that had to be shared, constantly reminding me that great things take time and they are often tackled day by day. Think progression and not perfection and I can assure you everything else will follow.

I'd like to thank everyone who supported me in this endeavor and especially those who took the time to read and critique the book before it was finished. Specifically I'd like to thank Nick Witzack, my business partner and true friend, for always being there to solve any problems I came across and being more than willing to help, as well as the number one person in my life who I know will always tell it like it is, Jaqueline Favaro, for constantly pushing me through the most difficult step in my project, starting and feeding the engine of motivation in me throughout. I appreciate you all.

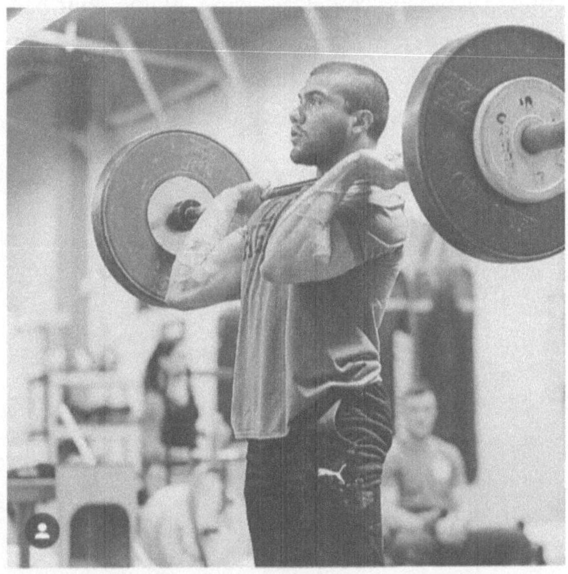

My introduction into health and fitness was the result of going through many phases throughout my life: the chubby kid growing up, one of the smallest of my friends, and even going through a brief phase of anorexia as well as bulimia.

After years of working out, the excitement that came with exercising slowly dissipated and the gym became a chore. On the brink of giving up working out altogether and finding another hobby, I discovered powerlifting, which reinvigorated that fire once again. It was an honest sport. Progress was tangible. It was black and white; you were either stronger overtime or you weren't. Competing soon followed, and some first-place victories along with it.

As with anything, if you want to grow, you need to have an open mind to everything. Having dabbled with a bit of Olympic weightlifting and satisfied with what I've accomplished in powerlifting, my next goal is to step into the world of competitive bodybuilding to keep the fire from going out and more importantly to broaden my knowledge of training and nutrition so that I can better service my clients and take my personal and online coaching business to the next level.

Health and fitness has opened up many doors for me, and I am grateful to the many people I've encountered (especially the ones I've trained) along the way. I've learned a bit from each and every one of you and because of that, you've all had a hand in my success.

PREFACE

This book came to fruition during the self-isolation requirements imposed by the Canadian government during the COVID-19 pandemic. The time which we once possessed, the majority of which was consumed by working and studying, was now spent at home, under isolated quarantine constraints. Being bored and having all the time in the world with my thoughts under those isolated conditions was the catalyst that sparked the creation of this book.

This is a health and fitness-related guide that focuses primarily on nutrition. This guide is for the newbie, the recreational lifter, the gym rat and the more serious athlete. I believe everyone from all ranks of experience can learn something from the following information throughout this guide. By no means do we dive into the vast complexities and scientific methods associated with each topic, rather a simple skimming of the surface to get a general overarching view of the entire picture. The guide is written in a way so that it is easy for any reader to digest. This book merely introduces you to topics and only goes so far into explaining things simply while using practical examples and anecdotal experiences with clients to facilitate the reader's understanding. If you can imagine two strangers sitting down discussing training and nutrition over a cup of coffee, this book will make a lot more sense.

The most difficult part of the writing process was deciding how in-depth I wanted to take each topic; finding the right balance of how much information to include and omit but still making sure everything made sense and included just enough detail. This book will introduce and/or have you revisit topics such as counting calories, structuring your own diet, dealing with cravings, coping with food during social outings and much more. I hope you enjoy reading it as much as I did writing it.

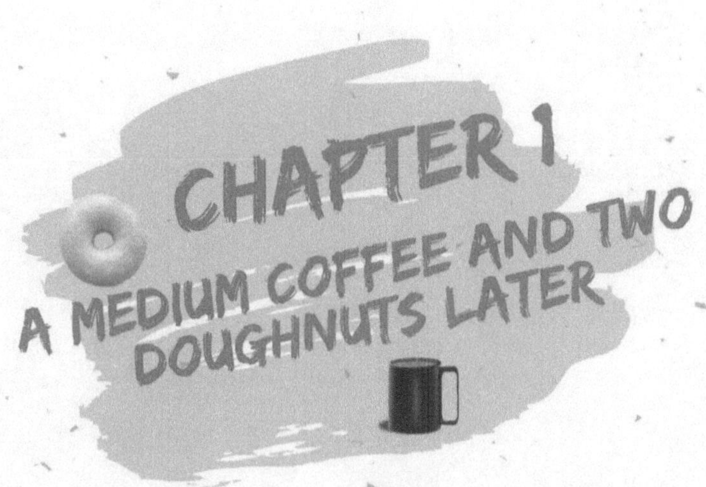

CHAPTER 1
A MEDIUM COFFEE AND TWO DOUGHNUTS LATER

1.1 COFFEE ANYONE?

It all began after I started offering online coaching services for training and nutrition. One service which I offer is monthly nutrition coaching. This is where I work with a prospective client on a weekly basis helping them to achieve their fitness and nutrition-related goals. I found that the easiest clients to work with were the ones who had a full grasp of flexible dieting (a method of dieting where clients keep track of their own food choices as opposed to following a rigid meal plan). The clients who were not informed about the principles of flexible dieting typically spent the first month of my services getting the hang of the concept, which wasn't desirable at either end, so I decided to offer detailed consultation services.

1.2 LET THE COFFEE COOL DOWN

The questionnaires I would send out before the consultations could only tell me so much, and oftentimes I would still find myself reaching out to clients to clarify what it is they meant. A potential client would reach out to me for help and I would send them a questionnaire and at the same time set up a date so we could go over it. It would either take place over the phone or in person. If the consultation happened in person, it would take place at either a Tim Hortons or Starbucks. I preferred Tim Hortons because they had doughnuts. The title makes sense now, doesn't it?

1.3 A CHOCOLATE DIP DOUGHNUT AND ONE ÉCLAIR

I would always buy a chocolate dip doughnut and an éclair (or a new flavor, if they didn't have it). I would strategically eat the doughnuts during the consultation while sipping on my own triple-triple – popular slang in Canada for ordering coffee with three creams and three sugars (I used three packs of sweetener and milk in my coffee). This left the person across the table from me always confused as to why I didn't just order a regular triple-triple. They would be even more taken back by the sight of me stuffing my face with doughnuts. It would always lead to the conversation of how I could get away with being "fit" while eating doughnuts. This was my time to shine! A couple of hours later, we would shake hands and I'd be off on my way, but not before grabbing another doughnut on the way out for the ride home.

CHAPTER 2

TELL ME ABOUT YOUR RELATIONSHIP WITH FOOD

2.1 ENERGY IN AND ENERGY OUT

Weight loss or gain, for the most part, is a game of numbers. How much energy do you expend versus how much energy do you consume? You can gain weight eating "good foods" just like you can lose weight eating "bad foods"; popular terms the health and fitness community like to associate with foods that contribute to fat loss/gain. There's a documentary called "Super Size Me" by Morgan Spurlock. It follows him on a 30-day period during which he ate only McDonald's food and gained a lot of weight (1).

There was also a movie called "Fat Head" by Tom Naughton. He also followed a McDonald's-only diet and not only lost weight but managed to improve his health markers after he had a blood test done (2). Strange, huh? Both documentaries were a little extreme on the diet, because nobody eats McDonald's every meal, every day, but it's in extremes that we can best get our points across.

There are is no such thing as "good" or "bad" foods. There are only those foods that will help you reach your goal more easily and those that will make it harder. The main message I want you to take away from this is that calories are king. Energy in versus energy out is what determines whether we lose or gain weight (fat and/or muscle) (3).

I've compiled a list of common training and nutrition practices and beliefs I've seen people come up with:

1. **Eating After 6pm Makes You Fat** – Why? Will a banana that is 100 calories at 5:59pm become 9,999 calories at 6pm?

2. **No Food Before Bed** – People choose not to eat right before bed because it's a period where they are not active. Bodily processes are still occurring, and this is a period

where your mind and body are under a state of repair during those hours of sleep. Feed it (4).

3. **Diet Soda Causes Cellulite** – I have no words for this. No one has successfully been able to explain to me the reasoning behind this statement. It's a case of broken telephone.

4. **I Cut Out Carbs** – Carbs always get the negative rap when it comes to the topic of fat loss. Bread is commonly the scapegoat. People are under the impression that carbs make you fat, so they cut them out. The weight lost that comes from cutting carbs is water (there is 2-3g of water in a gram of carbs) and having less glycogen (stored sugar in the liver and muscle) (5). The foods associated with gaining fat are typically those high in calories and carbs. By removing carbs from your diet, you're limiting your food choices and forgoing important nutrients found in food groups like vegetables, fruits, grains and dairy. For the sake of sounding like a broken record, you lost weight because 1) you are retaining less water and glycogen in the body 2) you've cut your grocery list extensively and as a result are consuming fewer calories overall.

5. **I Only Use Olive Oil, Never Cooking Oil** – Oil is oil. They all contain roughly the same number of calories per serving. Just because one is deemed healthier does not exempt it from its caloric content.

6. **I Have A Slow Metabolism** – No you don't. What you do have is the ability to underestimate the amount of food you are eating. Unless you have some sort of medical condition, the difference in your metabolism compared to someone else of your size might differ at most by a couple hundred calories. Even if you were to compare the metabolisms of small females with larger males, the difference is still only a few hundred calories (6). You can make up those few hundred calories by skipping that

frappuccino you usually get in the morning on your way to work. This BBC documentary gives great insight on how clueless people can be with their daily caloric intake and how most underestimate portion sizes of food: **"Do You Have a Slow Metabolism like this British Actress? See Shocking Test Results! | BBC Documentary"** (7).

7. **I Don't Want To Get Too Big** – This statement almost makes it seem like gaining muscle is so effortless that they have to catch themselves before they become a professional bodybuilder. It a tedious task that takes lot of time, patience and consistency. You don't have to worry about getting "too big, too fast".

8. **I Stopped Eating Meat** – So you've stopped eating meat and lost a ton of weight and now you feel better than ever. The reason for your weight loss comes from consuming less calories and food overall. You stopped eating meat and in doing so you also stopped eating the foods that are commonly paired with meat, if you were following the typical American diet. An example would be giving up eating burgers. No burgers means no bun, no condiments and no large fry and drink. Make sense?

9. **It's Healthier For You** – People like to create alternative recipes for foods deemed "bad for you" with healthier and higher-quality ingredients, such as recipes calling for honey instead of sugar or almond flour rather than white flour. Using higher-quality ingredients that contain more nutrients is just one part of the equation for being in good standing health. Having healthy levels of body fat and being at a healthy weight are other parts of the equation and sometimes these alternative recipes contain just as many, if not more, calories (which contributing to overall weight gain if eaten in excess) as the original recipe and taste much worse.

2.2 I'LL EAT WHATEVER AND GET THE BODY I WANT

Compared to whole foods, processed food has little nutrient value and is often high in salt, sugar and fat and although you can eat whatever you want and lose weight, there's a few reasons why you wouldn't want the bulk of your calories coming from them.

The first reason is you would potentially develop some sort of nutrient deficiency which could lead to health problems later down the road. Next, is that they are highly palatable, engineered in a way so you "can't have just one". Ever try having just a few chips? This leads to the last reason, which is that typically they aren't satiating enough, causing you to be hungry again shortly after having just eaten (8).

2.3 WHAT SHOULD I BE EATING THEN?

The hardest thing with dieting is always feeling hungry. Processed food is generally lower in protein and fiber, along with being low in nutrients (minerals and vitamins and trace metals) as I've mentioned before. What you want to be consuming are whole grains, fruits and vegetables, as well as animal protein; opting for leaner cuts as opposed to fattier cuts.

Imagine you're dieting and you spend more than half of your days' worth of calories on a single meal, early in the day. Now you have to spend the rest of the day walking on eggshells avoiding going over your calories. Picture this: in place of that one meal, you maybe could have eaten two or three sizeable meals of an animal protein with a serving of grains and vegetables and some fruit for dessert. It's a constant battle of needs and wants when dieting. Should you satisfy that craving that's bugging you, risking the chance of being hungry shortly after or forgoing it for the sake of satiety so that you can survive the hunger pains until your next meal? Choose wisely.

2.4 WHAT'S THE BEST DIET?

The best diet is the one that is convenient for you and you can sustain it long enough to achieve your goals. There's a higher chance you will follow it more than a diet that has been proven to be better than the one you chose to do, but you can't adhere too. Take the keto diet, for example. This diet works well for weight loss. Take a look at your current lifestyle right now and ask yourself this series of questions: could you cope with removing an entire macronutrient (in this case, carbs), avoiding vegetables, fruits, grains and dairy? Is this a diet you can sustain for the long term? Do you have the financial resources to be spending more of your grocery bill on animal protein? Is it an inconvenience for your friends or family every time you go out to eat?

2.5 YOU CAN HAVE YOUR DOUGHNUT AND EAT IT TOO

All diets work or can be tweaked to make work depending on your goal. That being said, I find a diet that includes a bit of everything and doesn't overly restrict one thing is generally the most sustainable. if you have a sweet tooth you feel you have to satisfy everyday just apply the Pareto principle to your diet: 80% of the foods you consume should come from a variety of food groups. It should contain fiber and adequate amounts of protein. The other 20% can come from your favorite processed foods, guilt free.

2.6 TO FLEX OR NOT TO FLEX?

As much as I dislike meal plans, they tend to work very well when clients can adhere to them. The meal plans I am talking about are the tried and true old school bodybuilding templates; the staples like chicken, rice, eggs, broccoli, oatmeal, white rice and so on. Eating around five meals a day spread three or so hours apart.

Well-structured and strict with not little room for flexibility for your processed foods. This type of eating structure shines when the goal is to step on stage opposed from just wanting to "look good naked".

The difference in the effort of the two is like night and day. Keeping that in mind, why do I dislike typical "bodybuilding" meal plans but at the same time praise them? There are many reasons but here are five major ones:

1. **A Better Outcome** – Weight loss is the goal for both dieting to "look good naked" and stepping on stage. When you're competing against others to win, the quality of the outcome matters; losing fat while maintaining the most amount of muscle. I find the quality of the food (especially protein) increasingly more important than just fitting anything into your diet to meet your caloric needs. An example would be opting for a chicken breast rather than a protein bar to reach your protein intake. Again, WEIGHT loss versus FAT loss.

2. **Higher Food Quality** – Being lean enough to step on stage requires a lot more effort with diet and nutrition. You will be doing A LOT more cardio and consuming A LOT less calories. It's unfortunate but it's what has to be done, and because you will be consuming low calories in conjunction with expending a lot of energy through exercising, you want to ensure that the foods you are consuming contain the highest amount of nutritional value as possible. Basically, it comes down to what foods you can get for the biggest bang for the buck. The buck in this case being calories.

3. **Consistency And Predictability** – Two important factors when It comes to dieting down to very low levels of body fat. Consistency here pertains specifically to food – your intake of calories and macronutrients.

Predictability has to do with knowing how your body will react in response to your food intake. This is important when prepping to step on stage because everything you do is for that one specific day. The farther you are into your diet, the less in the dark you want to be. If every day you're eating a different ratio of carbs, protein and fats then it will be harder to gage how your body will look on the day that really matters. With meal plans, every day you are consuming the same foods. There is no variability and there is 100% consistency and when changes need to be made in your diet, it can be done with relative ease and little guesswork.

4. **Satiety** – As I've mentioned before, to get stage ready, it will require suffering of all kinds, especially with always feeling hungry. Therefore, you need to include foods that are voluminous and contain very few calories. It will be difficult to diet to low levels of body fat while trying to eat processed foods as opposed to eating fruits, vegetables and animal protein.

5. **Avoid Food Cravings** – It's common to spend the entire day thinking about food when dieting. It's similar to if I told you to not think of the color red and now because I've told you, you can't stop thinking about the color red. The more we can't do something or the more restrictions we place on ourselves, the more we want to break the rules. If you let things slide once, it becomes easier to let them slide the more you do it.

The longer you diet and the leaner you become, the harder it is to make the right choices with your nutrition. A point will come where just a couple of chips isn't enough and even planning and fitting it into your diet can backfire. This can lead to a binging spree that comes from the mental fatigue and lack of energy due to having low levels of body fat and being in a prolonged deficit.

Trying to satisfy a craving can work early on, but it can also intensify it the deeper you are into a diet. The wise thing would be to avoid this situation all together and stick to the mundane foods for the longest time possible.

CHAPTER 3
ABCD...EAT, NEAT, TEF, BMR AND TDEE!

3.1 TOTAL DAILY ENERGY EXPENDITURE (TDEE)

Your TDEE is the amount of energy used by your body through movement and needed to keep the body working healthfully (9). It's not just a single measure, but is calculated as a sum of the following four forms of energy:

3.2 EXERCISE ACTIVITY THERMOGENESIS (EAT)

This is the amount of energy expended during exercise. It accounts for 5 to 15% of your total TDEE, the top end being relatable to athletes. It's not that much (10).

People seem to believe that exercising burns an absurdly large number of calories and in doing so they justify rewarding themselves afterwards by eating a lot. An example you've probably come across is going to All You Can Eat Sushi after an "intense" leg day.

You can expand a lot of calories through exercising but don't believe doing a few couple of sets for reps is going to cut it. It's going to require a lot more effort to earn that sushi. The difference in calories expended between the recreational lifter who exercises a couple of times per week for an hour compared to the athlete who does this for a living is large.

3.3 NON-EXERCISE RELATED ACTIVITY THERMOGENESIS (NEAT)

This is every other physical movement not associated with exercising. It includes your activities of daily living like maintaining posture, standing, sitting, fidgeting, walking to the refrigerator to grab that leftover cake from Karol's birthday, and many other unplanned movements (11).

NEAT is considered the most variable component of your TDEE and can fall between 15 and 30% of one's TDEE because it encompasses such a wide variety of activities. Take the person who works a sedentary desk job compared to the individual who works a job in construction. Who do you think uses up more energy throughout the day and who do you think will be able to lose weight on a higher number of calories? It isn't the person spending most of their day sitting down.

3.4 BASAL METABOLIC RATE (BMR)

Your basal metabolic rate is the amount of energy your body uses to keep you breathing and your blood flowing and constitutes 60-75% of your TDEE (12). It excludes the energy lost eating, exercising and performing daily activities not relating to exercise; basically, if you were to lie in bed all day.

Your body still uses up energy even if you aren't moving. What sort of activities are these? Thinking, breathing, digesting, etc. Keep in mind that muscle is metabolically costly whereas fat is not and therefore It uses up more energy. The same can be said for a heavier person compared to a lighter person. So, the more muscular and heavier the person, the more calories they expend at rest (13).

3.5 THERMIC EFFECT OF FOOD (TEF)

Your TEF is the amount of energy used to digest, absorb, and store nutrients from what you eat and drink. It's the form of energy that makes up the least of your TDEE, which can be up to 10% (14). You're probably thinking, why is there a range with TEF? Is there a difference in the speed or intensity applied to chewing and eating food?

The reason for the range is because protein is metabolically costly. It takes quite a bit of energy for your body to digest, absorb, and store it. Studies have shown that 30% of energy is used up by the body performing the bodily activities needed to survive. The energy wasted digesting, absorbing, and storing dietary fat and carbs is 2% and 8% respectively (15).

In a practical setting, this means that it can be harder to gain weight on a diet that's higher in protein than one that isn't. If Person A were to consume 1000 calories' worth of protein and Person B 1000 calories' worth of fat, Person A's intake would be less than that. Roughly 30% is lost through energy. Person B however would be intaking closer to 1000 calories (since 2% is energy wasted through bodily processes described above). This means that Person A in theory would need to consume more calories overall than Person B to reach that goal of 1000 calories. Have I confused you yet? I hope not.

CHAPTER 4
NUTRIENTS HAVE FEELINGS TOO

4.1 SCHOOL ME

Protein, fats, carbs and water are classified as macronutrients and are the nutrients that the body uses in relatively large amounts, hence the term "macro-". They are measured in grams. Micronutrients on the other hand are nutrients your body needs only in small quantities and the unit of measurement used is micrograms. These are your vitamins and minerals. We will be focusing on macros.

All foods are a combination of those four macronutrients. We will exclude water because it has zero calories and does not contribute to the caloric content of food. Proteins and carbs contain approximately 4 calories per gram and fat contains 9. When added, they should equate to the number of calories listed on a food label. For example: half a cup of oatmeal has 27g of carbs, 3g of fat and 5g of protein which if added should equate to roughly 150 calories.

27g x 4 calories + 5g x 4 calories + 3g x 9 calories = 155 calories

Just like some foods can be found to contain a combination of all the macronutrients, they can also be made up of only one or two of them; olive oil contains calories coming from fat only and a rib-eye contains calories coming from both fat and protein.

4.2 SKINNY MINNIE

What is the purpose of protein, carbs, and fat in a diet and how can you can apply them in yours? This section will be split into two parts: the first will focus on weight loss and the second on weight gain. Before we begin, I wanted to reiterate that calories are king. No matter the combination of macronutrients in your diet, you will not achieve weight loss or weight gain if your calories aren't controlled for, meaning if your goal is to lose weight, you have to be eating less calories than you are consuming, regardless of the breakdown of macros in your diet.

1. **<u>Protein</u>** – Extremely important the leaner you become. As a rule of thumb, the longer you are dieting for, and the more fat you lose, the more at risk you are for muscle loss. Muscle is metabolically expensive so the less your body has in times of starvation (forced in this case), the less it wants to hold on it. Having a diet that is high in protein can help mitigate that. Protein is also very filling. If you ever feel hungry while dieting, try increasing your protein intake.

2. **<u>Carbs</u>** – Your body's preferred source of fuel. Studies have shown that they have an effect on a person's mood and energy. This is why diets that cut out carbs completely can make people feel depressed, irritated, and lethargic. Lack of carbs can hinder one's performance depending on the type of training that is being done (16). Carbs are made up of three components: fiber, starch and sugar. Fiber and starch are complex carbs, while sugar is a simple carb. Simple carbs include refined sugars like soda, juice, and breakfast cereals. Complex carbs are high in fiber and digest more slowly. Main sources would include fruits, vegetables, nuts, legumes and whole grains. Starches can be found in the same foods as fiber like potato, rice and whole wheat bread. If hunger is an issue when dieting, try increasing your fiber intake as fiber slows down the digestion of food and can help regulate your insulin levels. Foods that are high in fiber are typically very voluminous in size and harder to overeat on. Taste aside, I would say it's a lot more difficult to consume large amounts of vegetables than it would be to consume a bowl of your favorite breakfast cereal, calories being equal. One will leave you constipated from all the fiber and the other in a sugar-induced comatose state.

3. **<u>Fats</u>** – Crucial for the production of sex hormones. Eating a low-fat diet can lower them. However, if your calories and body fat are low enough, your hormone levels will decrease regardless. Fat has also been shown to slow down the digestion of food (17). The key difference here is that carbs and proteins will fill you up during the meal because they will occupy space in your stomach. This will affect how much you can eat in one sitting. Fat on the other hand, because it slows digestion, can keep you fuller for longer between meals.

4.3 I WANT TO GET MASSIVE

On the other side of the coin, the three macronutrients' role if your goal is to add weight:

1. **<u>Protein</u>** – Protein is not as important when trying to gain weight as it is while trying to lose weight. Therefore it can be lowered because you will have a surplus of calories and most likely consuming higher carbs, both of which have a protein-sparing effect. This means your body will not pull protein from your skeletal muscles, converting its amino acids into glucose – a process called gluconeogenesis (18). If you have a poor appetite, a high-protein diet can be difficult to follow if you're trying to consume more food than you are accustomed to in order to meet your caloric needs, since it's the most filling of the macronutrients (19). For those wanting to minimize the amount of fat gained while trying to add on muscle, I find consuming a higher-protein diet than normal in conjunction with a slight surplus over a longer period of time is the best strategy. You need to find a happy medium where you are comfortably able to eat enough calories and protein to pack on quality weight (more muscle than fat), all while

trying to avoid gaining an unnecessary amount of fat in
the process.

1. **Carbs** – If your appetite is not the greatest, then I would
   advise you to limit the amount of complex carbohydrates
   in your diet and lean more towards simple sugars. Simple
   sugars typically take up less space per calories provided,
   preventing you from getting too full. Also, because they
   lack fiber, they digest much faster.
2. **Fats** – A great way to sneak in more calories into your
   diet since fat contains more than twice the number of
   calories per gram compared to protein and carbs. Foods
   that are primarily high in fat are typically small in volume.
   However, too much fat can slow digestion as mentioned
   before. Just like with protein, you need to find that happy
   medium that helps increase your calories but that doesn't
   affect your appetite much. To minimize the amount of fat
   gained while trying to add on weight, a lower-fat
   approach is recommended because its TEF is the lowest
   of the macronutrients.

4.4 NOT ALL BROTEIN IS EQUAL, BRO

A complete protein contains all of the essential amino acids our
body cannot produce on its own. Not all foods that contain
protein are complete and some contain higher ratios of amino
acids that are better for building muscle than others. Proteins
from animal sources are the most complete whereas legumes,
grains, fruits and vegetables are not (20).

The serving of protein waffles you had for breakfast might
contain the same number of grams of protein that a serving of
steak has, but not the same quality of protein. When you're in a
deficit, you only have so many calories to play around with. The
lower the calories, the more crucial it is that the food you're

eating is of the highest quality to ensure you are getting the most amount of nutrients as possible. Trying to meet your protein demands by eating things like protein bars, although not terrible, isn't optimal.

This is one of the arguments with going vegan or vegetarian. The claim is that they can meet the same dietary protein needs as with other diets that include animal products. They can. However, they would need to consume more overall protein because plant proteins are not as well digested and processed by the body as animal proteins and, because plant proteins are incomplete, they would need to include a greater variety of food sources that complement each other; an example would be combining rice with beans (20).

CHAPTER 5
YOU MIGHT NOT BE FLEXIBLE BUT YOUR DIET CAN BE

5.1 ADD SOME STRUCTURE TO YOUR DIET FOR F@$% SAKES!

First things first, you need to find your maintenance calories. This is the theoretical number of calories you need consume in order to maintain your weight given your current activity levels. The first thing is to go online and search for a calculator so that you can estimate your basal metabolic rate. There are various types online that you can use. None of them are entirely accurate, just estimates, and each type of calculator can slightly differ in calories from the next. The numbers given are just starting points. I prefer the one that uses the **Mifflin-St Jeor Equation** (21).

You input your height, weight and age. It will calculate your basal metabolic rate based on those inputs. You then take that number and multiply it by an activity factor provided on the website and this should be your maintenance calories, supposedly. To test this number, you would need to track it for around two to three weeks. The weight would be taken first thing in the morning after going to the bathroom. This would be done for span of seven days to find the average of the week. If your weight is stable in those weeks, that means you've found your maintenance calories.

5.2 IT'S THE SIZE THAT MATTERS

After finding your maintenance calories, you then need to determine the length of your diet. The shorter the length of the diet, the bigger the deficit can be and the higher your protein intake should be. The longer the diet, the smaller the deficit should be and the lower your protein intake can be (22).

The greater the deficit, the more at risk you are for losing muscle and the more disruptive it is to your body. To combat this, you would increase protein and shorten the length of the diet to help mitigate muscle loss and prevent you from hitting a roadblock too soon. Longer diets with smaller deficits in my opinion are better because not only can they better help to retain more muscle, but you also give yourself more time to form lifestyle habits needed to keep the weight off after losing it (22).

For gaining weight, a small surplus of calories every day over a long period is more advantageous than trying to pack on weight too quickly. The less fat you can gain trying to add muscle the less fat there is to lose, potentially shortening the duration of your diet when the time comes.

5.3 I WANT IT AND I WANT IT NOW!

If you're trying to gain or lose weight, the key thing to keep in mind is having your body functioning optimally so that most of the weight gained is going towards building muscle and most of the weight lost is coming from fat. Your body can efficiently do this when it is working optimally.

The goal of dieting is should be to lose as much fat while eating the greatest number of calories and retaining as much muscle as possible. When it comes to gaining muscle, it's best to avoid gaining too much fat because you want your insulin sensitivity to be high for the sake of nutrient partitioning (more of the food you digest goes towards building muscle rather than storing fat). The more body fat you put on, the easier it is to put on more fat (23).

5.4 NOW WE DIET

Now that you know your maintenance calories, the next step is to define your purpose for dieting and set goals. Once that's done, give yourself a time frame so that you can then determine your deficit or surplus.

1. The Cut

You've decided to cut (strip away body fat). Whatever your deficit may be, the process will be the same. You've tracked for three weeks and your weight has been stable so now you will need to lower calories to begin the weight-loss process. You do that and begin dropping weight. A week goes by and you lost an average of 2 lbs. Don't change anything. Another week goes by and you dropped an average of 1 lb. At the end of the sixth week you hit a roadblock and your weight stalls. Your first reaction might be to change something. DON'T. You need to first ask yourself a series of questions to determine why it was your average weight did not drop this week. These questions can be found in section 5.5.

If, after asking yourself those questions, you've found that none of them applied to you, then you can make a change. You have four options. You can wait it out for one more week because when you lose fat, fluid will temporarily enter and occupy the fat cells, and this is called the **"Whoosh Effect"** (24).

Let's say that's not the case and you still weigh the same after one week of waiting. You can either add some form of activity, decrease calories or implement a bit of both. You would add more activity if **1)** Your schedule allows for it, and **2)** Your appetite prevents you from decreasing calories any further.

With option 1, you might be wondering, wouldn't increasing my activity levels affect my appetite? Everyone's hunger response is different. Your hunger response to increased activity can be disproportionately higher compared to someone else's (25). An example would be how some people might be able to eat right after a workout while there are others who can't.

If your schedule does not allow you to increase your activity levels, then you would need to reduce your caloric intake. Another reason to reduce your caloric intake is if your hunger levels are fine. Reducing calories is a more certain way of ensuring weight loss compared to increasing your activity levels. Eating 100 fewer calories per day takes less effort than having to expend that many calories through exercise. Also, the calories tracked on cardio equipment as well as fitness devices are not entirely accurate and are only estimates.

How low should I decrease my calories and by how much should I increase my activity levels? This depends entirely on the goal you've set for yourself. I like to decrease calories by 10% and activity by ~30-45 minutes a week. If I am doing a bit of both then I would decrease calories by 5% while increasing my activity levels by ~15-30 minutes per week. These are rules of thumb. Lastly, when decreasing calories, try to never lower protein and always take calories away from carbs and/or fat. If anything, protein always goes up, especially the leaner you are.

As for how much weight you should be losing per week, another rule of thumb is, the leaner you get the lower the percentage of your bodyweight you would want to lose. Weight loss should slow down the leaner you become. I would be ok with clients losing between 1-2% of their bodyweight if they are above 15% body fat. If between 10-15% I would aim for 1% of their bodyweight and if less than 10% I would not try to lose more than 0.5%. If a client is 20% or above I would aim for more than 2%. Once again, these are rules of thumb.

2. The Bulk

You're done with your weight-loss phase and now you decide it's time to add on some size. Although the goal is different, the process is the same. You would calculate your new maintenance calories. Why new? If you dieted right, you should be lighter, and a lighter body takes fewer calories to maintain.

To gain weight you have to eat in a surplus. How much? Again, that entirely depends on your goal and the time frame you've given yourself to get there. As I mentioned earlier, the slower you add weight and the smaller the surplus, the less fat you can potentially put on, and the longer you can bulk for before your body becomes insulin resistant.

How close you are to your genetic potential will dictate how much size and strength you can gain. Everyone's body will differ due to genetics. With my clients, I try to never steer too far away above 15% body fat. Once we reach that body fat percentage it's time to pull back on the surplus. The higher your body fat the higher the risk of becoming insulin resistant and that's not a favorable environment for your body to be in to efficiently put on muscle. You should always try to maintain some visibility in your abdomen (everyone's fat distribution is different – be aware of where you tend to store fat and use that as a marker of when to pull back).

If your weight stalls, before changing anything, ask yourself the same set of questions you would when dieting. If you find that none of them apply to you then you have four options. Wait it out another week to see if your surplus is adequate. The second is to reduce your activity levels. You would do this if you can't stomach the idea of eating more food. Less energy expended requires less food. The third option is to consume more food. The higher calories you can gain weight on while still keeping relatively lean is always a good sign as you will be consuming more nutrients to support muscle growth. The last option is to increase calories and lower activity. I would increase calories by 5-10% and lower my activity levels by 20-45 minutes per week, the lower end of the range when choosing option 4 and the upper end when going with options 2 or 3 respectively.

For those of you who have a small appetite this where calorically dense foods can help push your calorie intake up. Use them sparingly because an over-reliance on this approach can affect your digestion. Your calorie intake is high so you eat processed food to help you reach that calorie intake, but in doing so you can't digest the food properly so now your appetite is worse off than before. Familiar with the paradigm "I need the experience to get the job, but I need a job to have experience"?

A good strategy is to have your cheat meal be the last meal of the day, so it doesn't potentially get in the way of you being able to eat your other meals, since all you will be doing is eating and going to bed soon after. I would first try to tweak your nutrition, messing around with your macronutrient ratios, moving around certain meals or maybe try replacing certain foods with others before turning to processed food for the solution. Remember, it's not how much you can eat but rather how much you can digest, and processed foods can negatively affect your digestion.

5.5 WEIGHT LOSS STALL QUESTIONS

1. Did you weigh yourself going to the washroom?
2. Did you wake up at the same time to weight yourself?
3. Was your last meal before bed solid or a liquid?
4. Was your last meal before bed bigger or smaller than usual?
5. Did you exercise close to bed?
6. Was your sodium intake higher this week compared to last?
7. Was your water intake more or less the same this week compared to last week?
8. Are you on your period?
9. Did you introduce or remove any new PEDs or supplements?
10. Were you consistent with your training, cardio, and nutrition?
11. Was this week more or less stressful than your last?
12. Was your sleep pattern the same?
13. Was your step count as consistent as last week?
14. Did you do any outdoor extracurricular activities that would have you moving that you did not do last week?
15. Is your job physical and if it is, did you work the same amount of hours/days like last week?

5.6 THE JACK OF NO TRADES AND A MASTER OF NONE

Possibly the most desired goal in the health and fitness industry is losing fat and gaining fat-free mass at the same time, commonly known as the "repartitioning effect". It's possible but difficult to execute and especially true for highly trained athletes (professional bodybuilders) due to the law of diminishing returns. Gaining weight requires a caloric surplus while losing weight a caloric deficit, which removes the necessary fuel for anabolism (the building up of something; muscle in this case) (26).

The closer they are to having maximized their genetic potential the more effort is required with their training and nutrition to elicit new muscle growth (27). At this point in their "training career", spreading themselves too thin trying to achieve both outcomes could work against them and most likely lead to a stall in progress or, even worse, risk losing muscle. Don't try to be a jack of all trades. Don't chase to many goals at once, it's a sure way to get nowhere fast.

In a lot of cases, what people think they witness or experience isn't the repartitioning effect but rather what is actually happening is that by gaining new muscle, they only appear to look leaner because there is more surface area the fat has to spread over. The more muscle you gain, the more noticeable it is. If two identical people contain the same amount of body fat, the one who is more muscular will appear to look leaner. Other factors that can dissuade the appearance of body fat on one's body are fat distribution, muscle insertions and height. A few pounds of muscle or fat will look different on a taller person than it would on a shorter person.

That being said, the repartitioning effect is common not only in untrained individuals but also in those who are inconsistent with training, getting back into it, carry a lot of excess fat, are switching to different training regimes and those who use performance-enhancing drugs.

1. **The Beginner Bunch** – This group can just look at weights and see progress. Any small sort of stimulus will produce results because the body is so hyper-responsive and far away from its genetic strength and muscular potential. Ever hear the term "beginner gains"? It's real. (28)

2. **"The Routine Hopper" Bunch** – This group might have maximized what they can from one current style of training, but they can still continue to see progress if they switch to another style that provides a different stimulus. I can use myself as an example. I trained for powerlifting for longest time. At the time I was focusing on maximal loads, training in the lower rep ranges, and doing minimal exercises and volume outside of the core exercises I had to do for competition purposes. My growth was limited, or so I thought. Once I switched over to bodybuilding, training more frequently, doing higher reps, more importantly training the "muscle" and not the "movement", my physique improved a lot more than I had expected. As tacky as it sounds, there's something to muscle–mind connection. (29)

3. **The "Bro, What Do You Take?" Bunch** – This is the bunch that use performance-enhancement drugs. These drugs can enhance the chemical processes in the body making it a much more efficient machine, if used correctly, greatly speeding up the process of gaining muscle and especially retaining it while in a deficit than your body ever could under natural circumstances. It's like "beginner gains" all over again. (30)

4. **The "I'm Not Fat, I'm Big Boned" Bunch** – Due to the large number of calories stored for energy in the form of excess body fat in overweight people, they can

effectively lose fat while in the process of trying build muscle. (31)

5. **The "If Inconsistency Were A Skill" Bunch** – This is that friend who will go hard for two weeks then fall off, then be back at it a few months later because "summer is right around the corner", so they have to get "toned". They haven't stuck to training consistently enough to see any meaningful changes that will stick, so they usually just give up when they figure out it requires more effort they are willing to put in. There is still a lot of room to grow for them since training nor nutrition was maximized long enough. Believe me when I say that you will see greater results being on the worst program if you are consistent with it, than the person on the best program who isn't consistent. (32)

6. **The "Just Getting Back Into It" Bunch** – Remember the old adage "It's like riding a bike, you never forget"? The same applies with training. If you've gained an appreciable size of muscle and strength, heck even the smallest amount, and stopped training for whatever reason, it's easier to gain it back again. This phenomenon is called "muscle memory". The response to training will be almost like that of "beginner gains". However, the older you are the harder it will be to get back to where you previously were. It takes a lot more effort to gain muscle then to maintain it. (33)

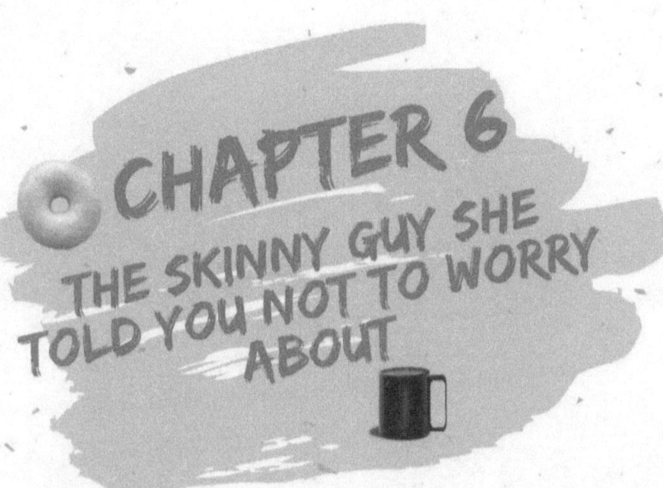

CHAPTER 6
THE SKINNY GUY SHE TOLD YOU NOT TO WORRY ABOUT

6.1 I GAINED IT ALL BACK!

Losing weight can be difficult, and so is keeping the weight off. The latter is a result of following a diet blindly without understanding why, in my opinion. People are looking for immediate results. I find taking a slower approach to dieting, giving yourself more time to lose weight, is a better approach because it gives you enough time to acquire the healthy lifestyle habits that will allow you to keep the weight off once you've lost it. Good habits can take time to develop and fad, crash, fast or whatever diets rob you of that opportunity.

6.2 MOTIVATION SUCKS

The problem is that people rely on motivation to keep them going, which I believe is an energy source you shouldn't rely on. You've probably witnessed it before, maybe even went through it. You'll get excited about a new endeavor like working out, so you buy the best training gear. You decide to tackle many goals at once. Before you know it, your progress comes to a halt and you get frustrated and burn out. As a result, you quit and return to your bad habits.

The secret is to take things one step at a time. Look for the low-hanging fruit. Take the little victories. This will help build your confidence and get you ready to take on bigger challenges. Doing it this way takes that extrinsic motivation you had for the gym and turns it into an intrinsic one, which has been found to last longer.

6.3 HABIT YOU LEARNED YET?

As mentioned earlier, good habits can take time to galvanize. When do you know you've formed a good habit or rid yourself of a bad one? Until it's no longer a second thought. When you don't have to waste "mental energy" thinking about it, you do it. An example would be not taking your shoes off every time you come home. Your significant other scolds you so you decide to kick this habit. At first, when you open the door to your house you will have to catch yourself. This is that mental energy I was talking about. The more time you repeat the task the more likely you are to open the door and automatically take your shoes off without even thinking about it. You have conquered the habit. Now you can move onto another one.

6.4 THE SINS OF THE OVERWEIGHT

Continuing on the topic of conquering habits. The same can be done with dieting. If someone who was overweight came to me for help, I would most likely not get them to do something as complicated as counting calories. That requires time to learn and quite a bit of effort. Remember, "low-hanging fruit".

Below is a list of common habits and poor lifestyle choices that can contribute to weight gain:

1. **Drinking Your Calories** – Not very filling and easy to overconsume. A cup of juice is 120 calories or so. No one drinks one cup of anything. If you have the habit of drinking something with every meal, you can easily be adding hundreds of calories a day to your diet.
2. **Cooking Oils & Butter** – A tablespoon of oil contains 120 calories and the same goes for butter. It's very common to use oil or butter in recipes and, in doing so, increasing the caloric content of whatever you eat way up. I would rather eat more of something that is solid, filling me up more, then eating less of it because I used cooking oil.
3. **Nibbles And Bites** – This includes everything from

tasting other people's foods, passing by the kitchen on the way to your room and grabbing a handful of trail mix that's out on the kitchen island, and licking the leftover Nutella on the knife after making a sandwich. These things add up.

4. **Snacking** – Eat a proper meal. Stop hoarding calorically dense foods in your desk drawer at work or in your car. If you can't kick this habit, then opt for lower-calorie snack options.

5. **I Put That S#@! On Everything** – Mayonnaise on sandwiches, ranch on salad, barbeque sauce on meat. Sneaky calories that don't provide much in satiety and just contribute to your total caloric intake for the day.

6. **Not Fidgeting Enough And Getting Distracted Too Easily** – Some people easily get distracted with tasks and they often forget to eat. Try to be like them. Constantly getting up and walking around and talking with your hands and keeping your mind occupied with tasks. The energy expended, however little, adds up over time.

7. **Eating Too Much In One Sitting** – This doesn't matter if you haven't gone over your caloric intake needed to maintain or lose weight. For some, spacing their meals to keep hunger at check throughout the day works, for others it doesn't. It's a bummer to eat all your calories early in the day and now you have to basically starve yourself the rest of the day. I've found that gorging on big meals can stretch your stomach, which can make it harder for smaller-sized meals to satisfy you. Have you ever starved yourself all day because you knew you were going to an all-you-can-eat buffet and when you finally got there you could barely eat anything (34)?

8. **Eating Out** – Dangerous. Restaurant food is meant to be delicious so that you can become a repeat customer. They could care less about your diet. More often than not restaurant food is jam-packed with cooking oils, butter

and sauces, pushing the caloric content of food that would otherwise be low, way up. That salad you ordered probably has more calories than the chocolate lava cake you decided not to have.

9. **Being Underactive** – Do you play sports or do your hobbies include reading and/or playing video games? Do you work a physical job or is it a sedentary one? Are you the type to stay home and watch movies when you're bored or go out for a nature walk?

10. **Halo Effect** – This is when someone overconsumes food because it is perceived or said to be healthy. Examples would be natural juice versus processed juice, organic versus non-organic, or protein bars versus chocolate bars, just to name a few. Because people think it's healthier, they think they can have more of it compared to its "unhealthier" alternative. Another good example is making "fit and healthier" versions of your favorite desserts when the original version tastes a lot better and at times contains fewer calories per serving. Here's a neat short video on the topic **"The Halo Effect (35)"**.

None of the things on the list require you to count calories. It's just a matter of choosing something from the list and conquering it until it becomes effortless to do. Once it has, pick another one or two things off the list and repeat the process.

I had this one client who came to me wanting to lose weight. After he explained his diet to me, I saw that a lot of the calories were in the form of liquids. He was from a tropical country so they were big on "natural fruit" and this ties in with the "halo effect" – because something is deemed to be healthy you think you can end up having more of it. I told them to continue with their diet but just to change one thing. Reduce or eliminate liquid calories (processed and natural juice, soda, milk, etc.) and instead replace those beverages with low-calorie, diet-friendly alternatives (diet pop instead of pop, or almond or 1% milk instead of regular milk). That client ended up losing 15lbs in one month, meaning that calories in the form of liquids were contributing to 15 lbs of their weight.

You might look at this list and realize that only a few apply to you. Heck, maybe none. If it is, then I doubt you're overweight and in that case the next step would be to start counting calories to get an idea of how much you are eating and go from there.

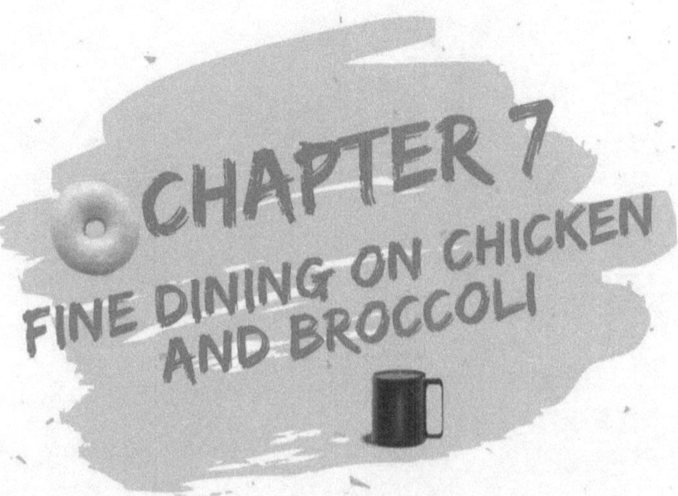

CHAPTER 7
FINE DINING ON CHICKEN
AND BROCCOLI

7.1 EATING OUT

It's annoying being on a diet and not being able to enjoy yourself when you're at some sort of event where food and/or alcohol are involved. Depending on how deep you are into your diet, you can still enjoy yourself. If you're on relatively low calories, then the strategies I'm about to share will be a lot harder to implement. Restaurants are notorious for their high-calorie dishes. You can easily consume over thousands of calories on a single entree and even more if you include the appetizer and dessert.

7.2 THE WORKOUT AROUND

Let's say that you are going to eat at a restaurant with friends and family. The first step is to find out which restaurant you will be going to and try to find their menu. Next, choose what you will be eating and track it using a food-tracking app of your choice (more on this later). By law, if a food establishment has more than 10 locations, they have to list the calorie content of what is on their menu (36). Mom & Pop-type restaurants will be a lot harder since there is never more than one of them. In the event you can't find what dish you are looking for at that specific food establishment, try to find something similar. An example would be eating at a Chipotle and being able to find the entry for their burrito versus a small burrito joint around the corner from your house.

The remaining calories are what you are left with to sustain you throughout the day until you get to the restaurant and so you need to control your hunger. To help with that, I would turn to things like zero-calorie beverages (coffee, diet soda, tea), chew on gum, eat a salad (avoid typical toppings) or lean protein. I would also leave some calories left over in case something unexpected happens and you end up eating more than you had planned for.

7.3 YOU'VE SURVIVED THE DAY. NOW WHAT?

As soon as you arrive at the restaurant and sit down, ask the waiter/waitress to remove the bread from the table. Either choose an appetizer or dessert. Ask the waiter/waitress things like how the food is prepared, to place the dressing on the side, for the cook to go easy on the oil or butter when cooking your food. Denny's is a perfect example of a food establishment that can make all of these necessary changes. Simple modifications like that could save you several hundred calories. Lastly, you don't have to eat everything on your plate, you can take it to go.

7.4 DAMAGE CONTROL

I will get more into the topic of tracking later on but let's say you couldn't control yourself and you ate more than you planned for despite your best efforts. There is always tomorrow. For the number of calories you estimated to have gone over, you could always mitigate the damage and reduce calories the next day or couple of days. If you went over your calories by 1000 on Friday, then you could eat 1000 calories less on Saturday or 500 calories less both Saturday and Sunday.

The same could be done with saving calories. If you find that the strategies I shared with you still wouldn't allow you to enjoy yourself then you could always save calories from previous days and add them on to the day you will be going out to eat. If you want an extra 1000 calories for Saturday and it's Monday, you could eat 200 calories less on Monday through to Friday and allot the calories you've accumulated throughout the week towards Saturday.

7.5 DON'T YOU DARE TOUCH PROTEIN

When reducing calories, especially when in a deficit, I try not to have my clients touch their protein intake. I usually pull away calories from fat and/or carbs. I like to keep protein as high as it can be. It's the most thermogenic and satiating of the three macronutrients and the most crucial for the recovery and retention of muscle (37). Again, all of these reasons become increasingly more important when in a deficit of calories.

7.6 MY FAVORITE MEAL IS ALCOHOL

On the topic of protein, I would take a different approach than the one above if your night out involves drinking instead of eating. Alcohol is detrimental to building muscle and for recovery but, more importantly, the dose is what makes the poison (38). If you know you will be going out to drink, the first thing is to track how many drinks you think you will be having. I would avoid drinks with sugar and stick to just hard alcohols. Also, I would consider beer over hard liquor since you can pace yourself whereas with shots you drink it in one go.

Next, try to eat more protein than what you would normally consume and lower fats and carbs to compensate for the increase in calories from the increased protein intake. Hydrate yourself well throughout the day, too. I would advise you to also give yourself a good number of calories for afterwards. People tend to make not-so-smart choices when under the influence of alcohol. Nothing tastes better than a late-night cheeseburger after a night of drinking and poor decisions. Am I right? Assume the worst and prepare for the worst.

CHAPTER 8
CHEAT CODES FOR "HELF"

Below are a list of habits and strategies that you can implement into everyday life to help you maintain (or lose) weight. A few of them will be familiar as they have been touched on previously in the book:

1. **Do Not Drink Your Calories** – Have the bulk of your calories come from solids rather than liquids. Solid food, for the same number of calories, takes up more stomach real estate which can leave you feeling more satiated than with liquid calories. If liquid calories aren't something you want to give up, then look for zero- or lower-calorie alternatives instead; such as replacing milk for almond milk or a soda for a diet one.

2. **Move More!** – Do more. Take the stairs. Walk. Bike. Play a sport. MOVE! Try to include some form of physical activity into your life outside the gym to increase your NEAT. The leaner you are the more your mind will subconsciously signal your body to move less throughout the day to offset the calories you burned exercising to conserve energy.

3. **Keep Busy!** – The busier you are, the less you think about food and the less time you have to sit down and eat. Fill your schedule up with things to do, keep yourself occupied and always be on the go! It's that simple.

4. **Food Environment** – Make it so that you are not around the foods that will make dieting difficult. Avoid buying triggers or remove them from out of sight. Instead of a bowl of nuts on the kitchen table, have fruits out instead; rather than using a clear jar for cookies, use one that isn't. Out of sight, out of mind, hopefully.

5. **Work For Your Food!** – The more effort it takes to

prepare or attain food the less likely we want it. Rather than having trigger foods out in the open, place them on the top shelf and out of reach, making it more of a hassle to attain them, which can deter you.

6. **Moderate These Foods** – Avoid or consume fewer foods that have been cooked or prepared with oil and butter, as this pushes up the calorie content of the food. The same goes with spreads, sauces, marinades, dressings and other high-calorie toppings. A naked bowl of vegetable salad is extremely low in calories but once you start dressing it with ingredients like olive oil, ranch, balsamic vinegar, cranberries, avocado and croutons you're looking at something that can potentially be hundreds or thousands of calories

7. **Plate Size & First Picks** – Keep small plates around. There is less room on it for food. If you want to take it one step further, make protein and vegetables the biggest visual component of the plate. Again, this will leave less room for potentially higher-calorie foods.

8. **Drink & Chew More** – Consume water before every meal as this will help with feeling full and with portion control. Coffee, being a stimulant, can help blunt hunger. Also, take the time to chew your food and eat slowly. Savor your food and the satisfaction that comes with it. Eating too fast doesn't allow the body the time to identify the satiety signals that develop before the end of a meal. (39)

9. **Always Overestimate** – If you aren't familiar with a particular dish or can't eyeball its calorie content, it's always better to lean on the safer side and overestimate.

10. **Meet Yourself Halfway** – Limiting processed foods and avoiding your favorite restaurant chains can be difficult. Instead of making changes to your diet with an all or nothing attitude, meet yourself halfway. There are a

couple strategies you could implement at first, before attempting these drastic changes. In the case of going out to eat, you could always make better decisions with your order. Simple changes like choosing grilled over breaded, chicken or beef and even choosing diet soda over regular is already a big step. You get to have your cake and eat it too. Another thing you could do, similar to the first, is look for healthier food establishments whose menus are more "diet friendly".

11. **Doggy Bag It!** – Remember, when eating out, you don't have to eat everything on your plate. If you are satisfied, ask to take the rest home.

12. **Meal Prep** – Planning your meals for the day will likely prevent you from making poor food choices on the fly. Even more so when you're really starving and the only thing on your mind isn't what can I eat that's healthy, but what can I eat to quickly satisfy my hunger.

Some of the above methods above can be a bit extra and, in some cases, ingrain certain negative behavioral patterns. For the general population looking for simple changes like improving health and losing a bit of fat, the above points can be applied mildly, so to speak.

What people need to understand, and often don't, is that to go the extra mile (i.e. the infamous six-pack), it takes a certain level of sacrifice that not many people can comprehend or are willing to put themselves through. Trying to diet down to low levels of body fat takes effort and can lend itself to obsessive and damaging practices. That's the nature of the beast.

For those who are more experienced with dieting, these methods laid out can potentially be useful when someone is taken out of their environment where they always have their meals prepped and a food scale on hand. Think of the above strategies as tools to help you stick to a plan when things start to go sideways; an unexpected family gathering, a night out drinking with friends or a vacation to an all-inclusive resort. Sometimes you just have to make do.

CHAPTER 9

THE MIND CHICO, IT'S A POWERFUL THING

9.1 IMAGINE THIS

You've cleaned up your diet. You took care of your home environment, meaning you took out all the trigger foods, so nothing tempts you during this weight-loss journey you've invested so much time, money, and energy into. The last thing you want is to come home, tired from work, and the first thing you see is a large order of pepperoni pizza and beside it a pint of Ben & Jerry's half-baked ice cream for dessert. No one in their right mind could resist that. I don't care who you are.

This is a predicament you do not want to be in. There's a workaround for everything, remember? The thing is the "cleaner" and the longer your diet the more tempting everything will be. There will come a point where you'll consider cereal as a dessert, and even rice will start to taste sweet. Let me introduce you to the diet brain.

9.2 BANG, BANG. I SHOT YOU DOWN

We all know it's not fun to just eat one cookie or a couple of fries or a handful of chips. Not only is it not fun, but it's not satisfying and it's a big tease. It will leave you wanting more, and the dangerous thing is, you will most likely have more. You think you can just tell yourself "Oh I'll have a few, or a couple of bites" and by the time you catch yourself, you've already eaten the whole thing.

Cravings don't go away easily. It's a persistent thought that will hunt you like that little robot dog-like thing in the *Black Mirror* episode "Metal Head", constantly in pursuit of its target. Until you deal with it, it will ruin you slowly, until you break. It's insidious like that.

9.3 LOSE THE BATTLE, WIN THE WAR

Decide for yourself that you WILL cheat. Yes, that's right, CHEAT! Decide what glorious mouth-watering food you will eat and on what day. Let's paint a scenario of how it would all pan out. There's an untouched box of Oreos your wife bought because you have kids at home and, well, they need to eat junk food too. Double stuffed. Goddamn it. To make things worse, Oreos are your trigger food. Get ready for a bit of math.

You know you can't have one and would be more than satisfied with eating 20 cookies. It says on the nutrition label 140 calories for two cookies. That means 20 would be 1400 calories. But wait! You know that you can't truly enjoy Oreos without at least two cups of milk. That's another 240 calories. Don't forget the two servings of Nesquik powder which is another 140 calories. After adding everything up, that's a whopping 1780 calories. You've decided on Saturday it's going down. It's only Monday, damn it! Now we wait.

9.4 LET THE CHEAT BEGIN

Saturday finally comes along. Your caloric intake to lose weight has been at around 2500 calories a day. You've strategically saved 200 calories a day to accumulate 1000 calories to add to Saturday. So, in actuality you've been consuming only 2300. Those 200 calories came from reducing carbs and/or fat. You did not touch protein. You have 3500 calories to put to good use for Saturday. You're the man.

You eat clean all day and night-time rolls around and you have your glorious cheat meal. You say "f@*5 it" and decide to have six more Oreos. But that's ok because tomorrow is Sunday and you can just eat 420 (70 x 6) calories less to compensate. Look at you. You did it. You killed your craving or that little robot dog from *Black Mirror* that's been chasing you.

9.5 YOU'VE EARNED THAT STOMACH ACHE

Now what? Now you go along with your diet as if nothing happened. Ignore the stomach ache and continue on with normalcy. You will hate life and you will be dying to get back on track with your diet. You most likely won't have another craving for weeks to come.

This is not something I would do frequently, only every now and then. It's much better to cheat this way, than to let your diet break you and have an unplanned cheat day or meal. This way you get rid of it while still being on track with your diet. You just have to deal with diarrhea for a couple of days, no biggie.

CHAPTER 10
BRING ME TWO MORE DOUGHNUTS

10.1 I DON'T HAVE CHICKEN. CAN I USE POP-TARTS INSTEAD?

As I've mentioned before, I dislike meal plans and so I try to avoid them when clients ask me for one. I'd rather teach a person to fish than to keep giving them fish. This is why I prefer a flexible dieting approach, because to be able to do it, some of the onus is on the client to learn how to measure, track and be more in tune with the nutritional labels of foods so that when the time comes to make trivial changes, they feel comfortable enough to do it themselves because they understand the "why".

More often than not, with meal plans, clients just blindly follow what you tell them to eat without asking questions as to "why". I understand that they aren't only paying for a meal plan but also to not be bothered with the nuisances of dieting. Some abuse this by constantly reaching out for any little hiccups: "I ran out of chicken, what can I use instead?", "Can I use brown rice instead of white?", "Does water have calories?"

Everyone needs to make money, but the true goal of a coach is to teach the client so that they can one day be able to do things on their own. It shouldn't be to always give them just enough information so they keep coming back and you can keep milking that cow. Teach, educate and let word of mouth do its job in bringing you income.

10.2 TRACK-MASTER-FLEX

Nothing frustrates me more than seeing a heap of tracking errors in a client's food log, especially when they tell you with all the confidence in the world "Don't worry, I've done this before". It's a bit of extra work but most of the time I'll get clients to add me on their preferred food-tracking app a couple of weeks before we begin just so I can monitor their tracking skills during that time. Any issues I see in their tracking, I'll correct them. That way we can work out all the kinks so that when we finally do start, the first month won't be a complete write-off from all the inconsistencies. After all, their results reflect on me as a coach.

Below is a list of the most common errors I've seen when tracking food. I will be focusing specifically on the tracking app called "MyFitnessPal" since it's the most popular and widely used. It's the one I prefer to use as well.

10.3 MOST COMMON TRACKING ERRORS (MYFITNESSPAL)

1. **I Want To Get A Divorce** – Track every single ingredient separately. If you are making a bacon, egg, and cheese omelet then track each one separately. Don't search for "bacon, cheese, and egg omelet". You'll find it, but it will be inaccurate.

2. **Always Go With McDonald's** – This might sound weird but bear with me. When you go out to eat and nothing is standardized, there's a greater margin of error. Let's use Chipotle as an example. Every burrito bowl can vastly differ in size depending on the person behind the counter making it. Some can be more generous and others not so much. If they woke up on the wrong side of the bed, then your burrito bowl might be smaller than usual, unfortunately. When it comes to places like McDonald's, every burger weighs essentially the same as the next, so tracking will be more accurate (40).

3. **Buff, Buff, Buff It Up!** – Continuing on with our Chipotle example, if you think the person behind the register overdid your order, meaning they were really generous then, in that situation, I would add an extra 10-20% calories more on top of what you tracked. It can be more or less, just whatever you feel comfortable with. It's better to be safer than sorry. If your order is

underwhelming then I would just track it normally because with dieting, it's always best to overestimate in situations like these.

4. **Take Me Higher** – Imagine you're over a friend's house having dinner and you did not bring your container of chicken and rice or food scale because that would not only be disrespectful, but they would most likely never invite you back. It's you, yourself and your terrible ability to estimate food. Don't fret, there's a way to mitigate the damage that might be done in this situation. The first thing would be to politely ask how the food was prepared and what ingredients were used. Next, try to find that food entry and choose the one with the highest number of calories. You survived the dinner and they might just invite you back.

5. **It's Complicated** – When eating out, try to pick dishes that are simple and easy to track. The more of the ingredients you can see, the better. It's less of a hassle to track an order of steak and potatoes than it is a fancy salad dressed head-to-toe. With the former, you will most likely know the cut of steak and the number of ounces but with the salad you'll spend most of your time figuring out how many tablespoons of dressing was used and whether they used a whole avocado or half; you might even start counting the cranberries sprinkled in.

6. **Don't Trust The People** – This might come as a surprise, but food entries listed on MyFitnessPal are user inputted, so be careful as some of them might not make sense. Make sure the macronutrients equal the calories listed on the nutrition label.

7. **It Won't Fit. That's What She Said** – Weigh your solids using a food scale and measure your liquids using measuring cups and spoons. I see this commonly done with peanut butter. My tablespoon is different from your tablespoon. And that difference could be a couple

hundred calories. Familiar with the phrase "heaping tablespoon"?

8. **I Put Detailed Oriented On My Resume** – Be specific when tracking food. Was the steak measured cooked or raw? What cut was it? Was the chicken breast braised, grilled, or baked? What brand was it? Was the rice long or short grain, basmati, or jasmine? 4 oz of raw skinless chicken breast is 125 calories whereas 4 oz roasted is 190 calories. That's a difference of 65 calories. If you were to make this mistake once a day, every day for a week, that's a total of 455 calories! Imagine if you were to make the same mistakes multiple times in a day. Be careful, it could mean a week's worth of dieting out the window.

9. **What They Don't Know, Won't Hurt Them** – Although including a variety of foods is good for a nutritiously balanced diet, it can make tracking more complicated. The more variety of food in your diet, the greater the margin of error there will be. Food companies are allowed a wide latitude in accuracy with the calories listed on package labels (20% in either direction); if something is listed as 100 calories, it could very well be 80-120. That's why being consistent with the foods you eat every day is a good countermeasure to bring you closer to your target calories. The inaccuracy in one food is balanced out by the inaccuracy of another and the smaller the margin of error will be. You have to find that medium of having enough variety to meet your nutritional needs while still being as accurate as possible with the number of calories you are consuming. Take a look at this by Casey Neistat done for the *New York Times* on the issue: "**Calorie Detective: The Real Math Behind Food Labels | Op-Docs | The New York Times**" (41)

10. **Good Ol' Homemade Apple Pie** – I would avoid the

"homemade" entries as those can be extremely inaccurate. Those are harder to cross-reference with other nutritional databases, like **www.calorieking.com**, in case you needed a second opinion in the calorie and macronutrient content of a food.

11. **Why 1+1 Does Not Equal 2** – With MyFitnessPal as well as other food tracking apps, you'll notice, if you haven't already, that the macronutrients almost never add up to the calories stated in your food journal. This is due to rounding errors. For a more thorough explanation be sure to watch Layne Norton's video on the topic, **"Why your calories and macros NEVER match"** (42)

CHAPTER 11
WE RAN OUT OF COFFEE

11.1 LOOK MA, WE MADE IT

Look at you, you've made it. You've finally read more than 10 pages in your life and not because you were told to finish some book reports for school but because you wanted to. Hopefully you've gotten as much out of this as my clients do during our consultations. Of course, don't just take what I said as the holy grail. Question and research everything that you might not agree with and goes against your way of doing things.

11.2 EXTRA! EXTRA! READ ALL ABOUT IT!

Stick to the tried and true. It works. Losing weight or gaining weight boils down to calories in and calories out. It's the nuances of dieting and your determination that lead to the quality of the outcome (macronutrient intake, meal timing, consistency, proper supplementation, cardio, etc.). It's in our nature to choose the path with the least resistance. What we want to see and hear is:

"Guaranteed weight loss in 10 days by drinking this special tea from the Brazilian Rainforest." Sound familiar? Or would you prefer *"Lose 10 lbs in 3 months! It will only take going to the gym 5 days a week and giving up eating junk food every day!".*

Simple and hard work does not sell, it's not sexy. Find a gimmick and you can almost certainly justify a high price for the service. Ridiculous, I know. It's just business at the consumer's expense, it's not personal.

11.3 RUN BRO, RUN!

Below are some common fitness gimmicks you might have come across or even fallen victim to at some point in your life. I know I have.

1. **Juice Cleanses/Detox** – Stop this. This is what your liver is for and it does this job very well. Avoid this gimmick at all cost. (43)

2. **The "So And So" Diet** – Avoid any diet that markets itself with having to buy some sort of gimmicky supplement for it to work. These diets work by getting the consumer to follow a meal plan that removes a whole food group or macronutrient, let's say carbs and maybe some specific food like bread, for example. Then they get the consumer to buy some expensive product like diet pills. There will most likely never be enough pills, so the consumer will have to keep buying more. The client follows the meal plan and loses 10 lbs in 10 days and is ecstatic. Little does the client know, some of that lost weight was fluid, reduced glycogen, and less food in their gut from the gastric emptying. Very little fat was lost! Now the client believes the weight loss was because of some special meal plan and magical bean stock pills. Not only that, but they swear off carbs and bread forever because they've been duped into thinking it's detrimental to fat loss.

3. **12 Minute Ab Workout for 12 Pack Abs In 12 Days For $12** – Any training program that promises fast and easy results, especially if it's sold along with some sort of gimmicky exercise equipment: avoid it like the plague. Just like with diet, the basics work. If you see something complicated, it's just a strategy to justify how expensive it is. Gaining muscle and losing fat is a marathon, not a sprint as clichéd as that sounds.

4. **The Perfect Meal Plan** – I've seen this plenty of times – a glorified meal plan that contains a bunch of "superfoods", useless supplements and the exact timing of when to eat the meals. If you're a healthy individual, the basics work. The problem is, you can't slap on a high

price tag. So, you throw in as many gimmicky things as possible to able to get away with doing that.

5. **Supplements** – The majority are overpriced and useless. The big pullers are the supplements that promise fat loss or muscle gain. If a supplement directly burned fat or helped with gaining muscle significantly, it could not be sold in a supplement store and would be considered a drug, in fact (44). More often than not, these supplements that promise these results are more expensive than the drugs themselves that actually produce these results! That's not to say you should avoid supplements altogether, but you should first have your training and nutrition in check first. The worthwhile supplements are the ones that will "supplement" the missing pieces in your training and nutrition and more importantly, your health: taking a fiber or a greens supplement in the meantime, because you find it hard to eat enough vegetables to meet the recommended daily amount, makes a lot more sense than going for something that promises to INCREASE MUSCLE MA$$ BY 30 LBS IN 7 DAYS!!!!!

6. **The Guru And The Internet Fitness Celebrity** – Remember, a lot of information you can find on the internet for free. So be extremely careful when shopping around for coaches. Look at that person's track record with clients, the reviews, how they market themselves and what their philosophy is with training and nutrition. With regard to fitness influencers, a lot of them, because of their following, give out cookie-cutter programs and meal plans to cater to the massive amounts of people reaching out to them every day. Don't be naïve into thinking you are getting something specifically catered to you or that it's in fact them responding to your email or text. Most likely it's someone in a different country who knows very little about

training and nutrition and is following a script. That booty blaster program for $99 isn't worth the risk, but then again, we learn best from making the mistakes ourselves as wise as it is to learn from other people's mistakes. There's emotion attached with the learning experience.

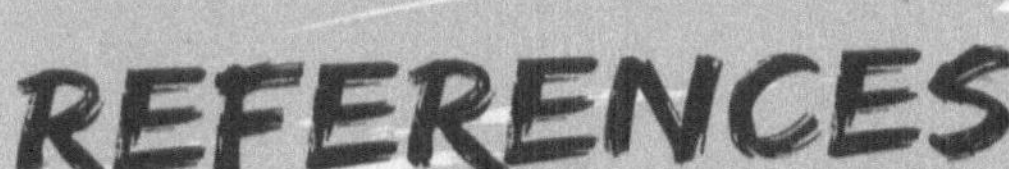
REFERENCES

1. Spurlock, Morgan. Super Size Me. New York, N.Y.: Hart Sharp Video, 2004.

2. Naughton, Tom. Fat Head. United States: Morning Star Entertainment, 2009.

3. National Research Council (US) Committee on Diet and Health. Diet and Health: Implications for Reducing Chronic Disease Risk. Washington (DC): National Academies Press (US); 1989. 6, Calories: Total Macronutrient Intake, Energy Expenditure, and Net Energy Stores. Available from: https://www.ncbi.nlm.nih.gov/books/NBK218769/

4. Kinsey AW, Ormsbee MJ. The health impact of nighttime eating: old and new perspectives. Nutrients. 2015;7(4):2648–2662. Published 2015 Apr 9. doi:10.3390/nu7042648

5. Oh R, Uppaluri KR. Low Carbohydrate Diet. [Updated 2020 Jan 3]. In: StatPearls [Internet]. Treasure Island (FL): StatPearls Publishing; 2020 Jan-. Available from: https://www.ncbi.nlm.nih.gov/books/NBK537084/

6. AskMayoExpert. Weight management (adult). Rochester, Minn.: Mayo Foundation for Medical Education and Research; 2018.

7. Video Source: BBC Documentary 10 Things You Need to Know About Losing Weight.

8. Hall KD, et al. Ultra-processed diets cause excess calorie intake and weight gain: A one-month inpatient randomized controlled trial of ad libitum food intake. Cell Metabolism (link is external). May 16, 2019.

9. Melanson EL. The effect of exercise on non-exercise physical activity and sedentary behavior in adults. Obes Rev. 2017;18 Suppl 1(Suppl 1):40–49. doi:10.1111/obr.12507

10. Melanson EL. The effect of exercise on non-exercise physical activity and sedentary behavior in adults. Obes Rev. 2017;18 Suppl 1(Suppl 1):40–49. doi:10.1111/obr.12507

11. von Loeffelholz C, Birkenfeld A. The Role of Non-exercise Activity Thermogenesis in Human Obesity. [Updated 2018 Apr 9]. In: Feingold KR, Anawalt B, Boyce A, et al., editors. Endotext [Internet]. South Dartmouth (MA): MDText.com, Inc.; 2000-. Available from: https://www.ncbi.nlm.nih.gov/books/NBK279077/

12. Trexler, Eric & Smith-Ryan, Abbie & Norton, Layne. (2014). Metabolic adaptation to weight loss: Implications for the athlete. Journal of the International Society of Sports Nutrition. 11. 7. 10.1186/1550-2783-11-7.

13. Metabolism and weight loss: How you burn calories. Rochester, Minn.: Mayo Foundation for Medical Education and Research; 2017.

14. Manuel Calcagno, Hana Kahleova, Jihad Alwarith, Nora N. Burgess, Rosendo A. Flores, Melissa L. Busta & Neal D. Barnard (2019): The Thermic Effect of Food: A Review, Journal of the American College of Nutrition, DOI: 10.1080/07315724.2018.1552544 To link to this article: https://doi.org/10.1080/07315724.2018.1552544Published online: 25 Apr 2019.

15. Barr SB, Wright JC. Postprandial energy expenditure in whole-food and processed-food meals: implications for daily energy expenditure. Food Nutr Res. 2010;54:10.3402/fnr.v54i0.5144. Published 2010 Jul 2. doi:10.3402/fnr.v54i0.5144

16. American Physiological Society (APS). (2015, December 15). Carbs, not fats, boost half-marathon race performance. ScienceDaily. Retrieved May 30, 2020 from www.sciencedaily.com/releases/2015/12/151215094542.htm

17. Ingram DM, Bennett FC, Willcox D, de Klerk N. Effect of low-fat diet on female sex hormone levels. J Natl Cancer Inst. 1987;79(6):1225–1229.

18. Kanter M. High-Quality Carbohydrates and Physical Performance: Expert Panel Report. Nutr Today. 2018;53(1):35–39. doi:10.1097/NT.0000000000000238

19. Noakes M. The role of protein in weight management. Asia Pac J Clin Nutr. 2008;17 Suppl 1:169–171.

20. Berrazaga I, Micard V, Gueugneau M, Walrand S. The Role of the Anabolic Properties of Plant- versus Animal-Based Protein Sources in Supporting Muscle Mass Maintenance: A Critical Review. Nutrients. 2019;11(8):1825. Published 2019 Aug 7. doi:10.3390/nu11081825

21. Journal of the Academy of Nutrition and Dietetics. Comparison of Predictive Equations for Resting Metabolic Rate in Healthy Nonobese and Obese Adults: A Systematic Review VOLUME 105, ISSUE 5, P775-789, MAY 01, 2005 DOI: https://doi.org/10.1016/j.jada.2005.02.005

22. Champagne CM, Broyles ST, Moran LD, et al. Dietary intakes associated with successful weight loss and maintenance during the Weight Loss Maintenance trial. J Am Diet Assoc. 2011;111(12):1826–1835. doi:10.1016/j.jada.2011.09.014

23. Liang, Xiongfei MD a,b; Chen, Xianhua MD b; Li, Jing MSc; Yan, Mengdan MSc; Yang, Yifeng MD a,* Study on body composition and its correlation with obesity, Medicine: May 2018 – Volume 97 – Issue 21 – p e10722 doi: 10.1097/MD.0000000000010722

24. Sissons, Beth. Is the whoosh effect real? Medical News Today. 2020. https://www.medicalnewstoday.com/articles/the-woosh-effect#what-is-it

25. Dorling J, Broom DR, Burns SF, et al. Acute and Chronic Effects of Exercise on Appetite, Energy Intake, and Appetite-Related Hormones: The Modulating Effect of Adiposity, Sex, and Habitual Physical Activity. Nutrients. 2018;10(9):1140. Published 2018 Aug 22. doi:10.3390/nu10091140

26. Am J Clin Nutr. 2007 85(4):1005-13. Resistance training and dietary protein: effects on glucose tolerance and contents of skeletal muscle insulin signaling proteins in older persons. Iglay HB, Thyfault JP, Apolzan JW, Campbell WW.

27. Ribeiro, A. S., Nunes, J., Schoenfeld, B. J., Aguiar, A. F., & Cyrino, E. S. (2019). Effects of Different Dietary Energy Intake Following Resistance Training on Muscle Mass and Body Fat in Bodybuilders: A Pilot Study, Journal of Human Kinetics, 70(1), 125-134. doi: https://doi.org/10.2478/hukin-2019-0038

28. Hubal, Monica & Gordish-Dressman, Heather & Thompson, Paul & Price, Thomas & Hoffman, Eric & Angelopoulos, Theodore & Gordon, Paul & Moyna, Niall & Pescatello, Linda & Visich, Paul & Zoeller, Robert & Seip, Richard & Clarkson, Priscilla. (2005). Variability in muscle size and strength gain after unilateral resistance training. Medicine and science in sports and exercise. 37. 964-72. 10.1249/01.mss.0000170469.90461.5f.

29. Baz-Valle E, Schoenfeld BJ, Torres-Unda J, Santos-Concejero J, Balsalobre-Fernández C (2019) The effects of exercise variation in muscle thickness, maximal strength and motivation in resistance trained men. PLoS ONE 14(12): e0226989. https://doi.org/10.1371/journal.pone.0226989

30. Bhasin, Shalender, Storer, Thomas, Berman, Nancy (1996). The Effects of Supraphysiologic Doses of Testosterone on Muscle Size and Strength in Normal Men. The New England Journal of Medicine. Massachusetts Medical Society.

31. Demling RH, DeSanti L. Effect of a hypocaloric diet, increased protein intake and resistance training on lean mass gains and fat mass loss in overweight police officers. Ann Nutr Metab. 2000;44(1):21–29. doi:10.1159/000012817

32. Hagstrom, A.D., Marshall, P.W., Halaki, M. et al. The Effect of Resistance Training in Women on Dynamic Strength and Muscular Hypertrophy: A Systematic Review with Meta-analysis. Sports Med 50, 1075–1093 (2020). https://doi.org/10.1007/s40279-019-01247-x

33. The amazing phenomenon of muscle memory. Oxford University. 2017. https://medium.com/oxford-university/the-amazing-phenomenon-of-muscle-memory-fb1cc4c4726

34. Gordon, Serena. Study: Body May Recover From Bursts of Overeating. American Journal of Physiology--Endocrinology and Metabolism. 2019. https://www.webmd.com/diet/news/20190513/study-body-may-recover-from-bursts-of-overeating#1

35. Wansink, Brian and Pierre Chandon (2006), "Can 'Low Fat' Nutrition Labels Lead to Obesity?," Journal of Marketing Research, 43 (4), 605-17. https://www.youtube.com/watch?v=ItBMVEvnrSc

36. VanEpps EM, Roberto CA, Park S, Economos CD, Bleich SN. Restaurant Menu Labeling Policy: Review of Evidence and Controversies. Curr Obes Rep. 2016;5(1):72–80. doi:10.1007/s13679-016-0193-z

37. Vliet SV, Beals JW, Martinez IG, Skinner SK, Burd NA. Achieving Optimal Post-Exercise Muscle Protein Remodeling in Physically Active Adults through Whole Food Consumption. Nutrients. 2018;10(2):224. Published 2018 Feb 16. doi:10.3390/nu10020224

38. Duplanty, Anthony A.; Budnar, Ronald G.; Luk, Hui Y.; Levitt, Danielle E.; Hill, David W.; McFarlin, Brian K.; Huggett, Duane B.; Vingren, Jakob L. Effect of Acute Alcohol Ingestion on Resistance Exercise–Induced mTORC1 Signaling in Human

Muscle, The Journal of Strength & Conditioning Research: January 2017 – Volume 31 – Issue 1 – p 54-61 doi: 10.1519/JSC.0000000000001468

39. Paddock, Catharine. Two Cups Of Water Before Each Meal Enhanced Weight Loss In Clinical Trial. Medical News Today. 2010. https://www.medicalnewstoday.com/articles/198720#1

40. Tarantino, Olivia. 30 Crazy McDonald's Facts That Will Blow Your Mind. Eat This, Not That! 2018. https://www.eatthis.com/mcdonalds-news/

41. Kluger, Jeffrey. Dieters Beware: Calorie Counts Are Frequently Off. TIME. 2010. http://content.time.com/time/health/article/0,8599,1951798,00.html

42. Holwegner, Andrea. Why your calorie counting apps and devices may be wrong: Fitbit and MyFitnessPal Issues. Calgary Herald. 2019. https://www.healthstandnutrition.com/calorie-counting-apps-devices-wrong/

43. Juicing -- Fad or Fab? Harvard Health Publishing. 2015. https://www.health.harvard.edu/healthy-eating/juicing-fad-or-fab

44. Collins, Francis. Study Finds No Benefit for Dietary Supplements. NIH.gov. 2019. https://directorsblog.nih.gov/2019/04/16/study-finds-no-benefit-for-dietary-supplements/